# HOW TO BE A
# FIT BIRD

## MARION DEUCHARS

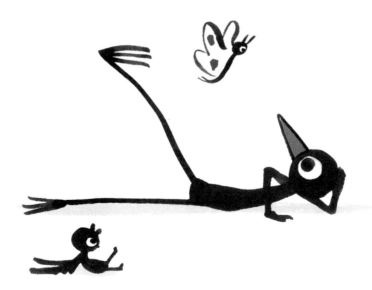

**§ Skittledog**

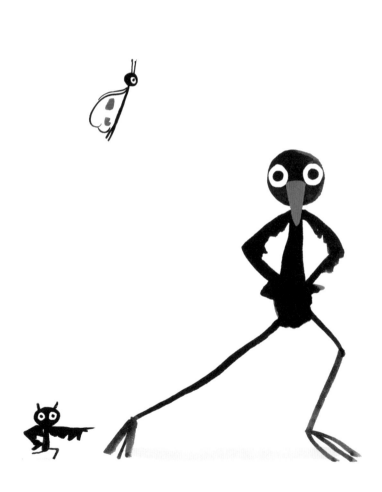

# FOREVER FIT

I used to be someone who stuck to low-impact exercise, which felt good but never really got my heart racing. However, after finding myself getting out of breath climbing the stairs or running to catch the bus, I realised it was time for a change. No big aims, no targets or weight loss — just a decision that exercise would be something I try to do every day, forever.

It's not enough to just want to live long: I want to live long and live well. I want to bend down and pick up a flower — and not fall over. I want to have enough energy to take on new things and I want to feel strong.

I hope this book will help you begin your fitness journey. It's for all ages and all abilities and it's never too late to start exercising. Doing something is better than doing nothing at all.

# EQUIPMENT ESSENTIALS

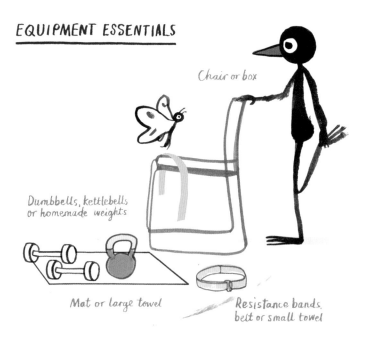

Chair or box

Dumbbells, kettlebells or homemade weights

Mat or large towel

Resistance bands, belt or small towel

# CONTENTS

THE SEVEN FUNDAMENTAL MOVEMENTS 7

EXERCISES FOR FLEXIBILITY & MOBILITY 21
⏱ WARM-UP 28

EXERCISES FOR CARDIO 31
EXERCISES FOR CORE 41
⏱ CARDIO & CORE WORKOUT 54

EXERCISES FOR LOWER BODY STRENGTH 57
⏱ WORKOUT 68

EXERCISES FOR UPPER BODY STRENGTH 71
⏱ WORKOUT 82

⏱ FULL-BODY WORKOUT 84

⏱ COOL-DOWN 86

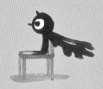

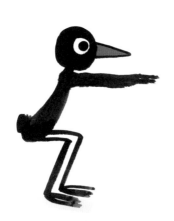

## 1. SQUAT

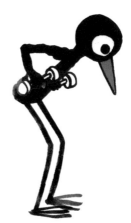

## 2. PULL

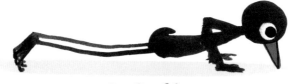

## 3. PUSH

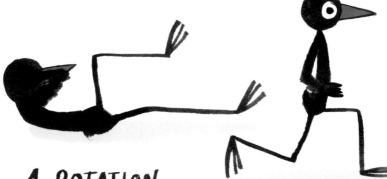

## 4. ROTATION

## 5. LUNGE

# THE **SEVEN** FUNDAMENTAL MOVEMENTS

These basic movements mirror our everyday activities, like carrying groceries, opening doors or reaching into a cupboard. But they also form the key part of many exercises in this book.

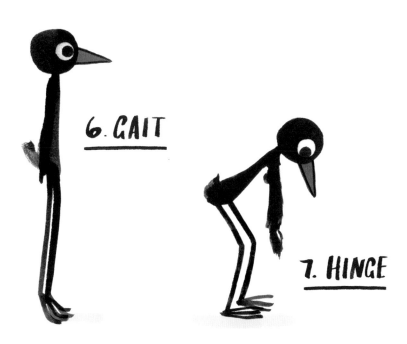

## 6. GAIT

## 7. HINGE

# 1. SQUAT

Squats target large muscle groups in the thighs, buttocks and lower back. Doing them regularly will make you feel stronger and help with mobility.

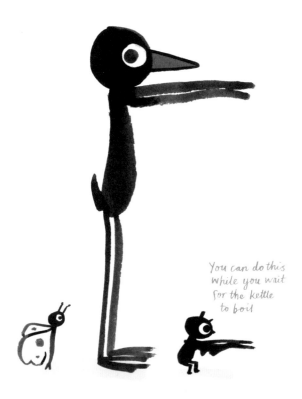

You can do this while you wait for the kettle to boil

# BASIC SQUAT

HEAD UP, NECK IN LINE WITH
SPINE, FEET HIP-WIDTH APART.
BEND KNEES, MOVING HIPS AND
BOTTOM BACK AS IF TO SIT DOWN.
KEEP KNEES OVER TOES. STAND UP,
SQUEEZING BUTTOCKS.

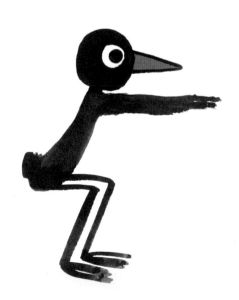

# 2. PULL

Pulling weights towards you targets your back, shoulders, upper arms, forearms and hamstrings. Pulling and pushing gives a balanced workout.

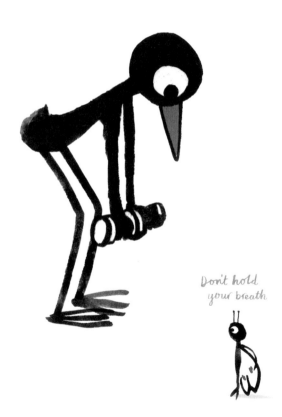

Don't hold your breath.

# BENT-OVER ROW

HINGE AT THE HIPS WITH A
FLAT BACK. HOLD DUMBBELLS
AND EXHALE AS YOU PULL
YOUR ELBOWS BACK. INHALE
AS YOU LOWER. REPEAT.

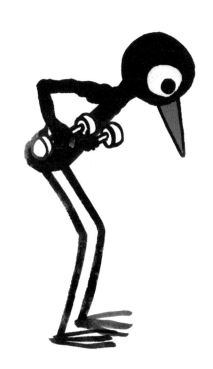

# 3. PUSH

Pushing weights with the arms targets the chest, shoulders and upper arms. Done with the legs, it trains the entire lower body.

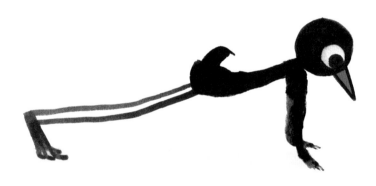

# PUSH-UP

WITH HANDS SHOULDER-WIDTH
APART, EXTEND YOUR LEGS BACK.
BODY STRAIGHT, HEAD IN LINE
WITH SPINE, LOWER CHEST TO
THE GROUND, ELBOWS TUCKED,
THEN PUSH UP. REPEAT.

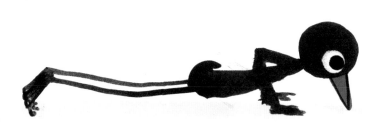

You can do
this on your
knees too

# 4. ROTATION

Rotation exercises involve twisting movements, mainly with the torso. Doing twists will make your body more agile and help with everyday tasks and sports.

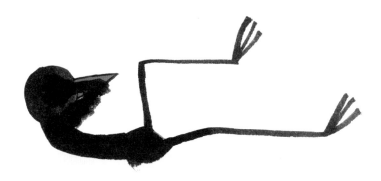

Alternate sides as if pedalling a bike

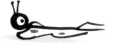

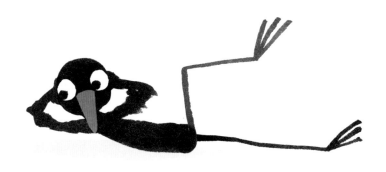

# BICYCLE CRUNCHES

LAY ON YOUR BACK, HANDS
BEHIND HEAD, LIFT SHOULDERS
AND BRING ONE KNEE TO
THE CHEST. TWIST THE
OPPOSITE ELBOW TOWARDS
IT. CHANGE LEGS AND REPEAT
WITH OTHER ELBOW.

# 5. LUNGE

Stepping forwards, backwards or sideways with one leg shapes and strengthens your lower body, also helping with balance and flexibility.

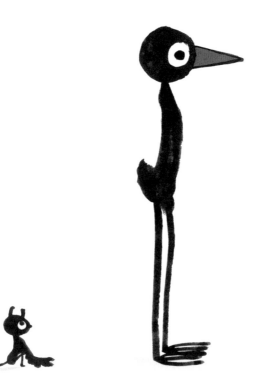

# FORWARD LUNGE

STRETCH RIGHT LEG BACK,
LEFT KNEE BENT AT A
RIGHT ANGLE. PLACE
HANDS ON HIPS OR BY
WAIST. DROP THE OTHER
KNEE TO THE FLOOR.
CHANGE LEGS AND REPEAT.

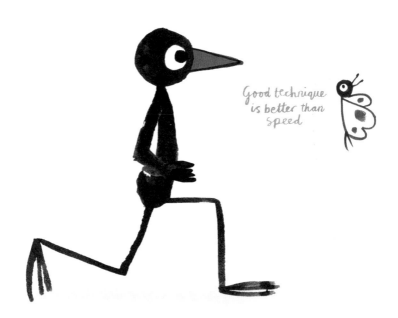

Good technique
is better than
speed

# 6. GAIT

Gait exercises help to strengthen your muscles; improving stability, mobility and the way you walk and run.

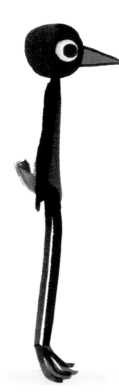

## TOE WALKS

STAND UPRIGHT, LIFT HEELS OFF THE GROUND, BALANCE ON TOES AND WALK FORWARD, MAINTAINING BALANCE.

Tippy toes

# 7. HINGE

Bending at the hips while keeping the back straight is called a hinge movement. It targets the back, buttocks and hamstrings.

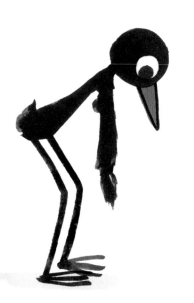

## DEAD LIFT

STAND WITH FEET HIP-WIDTH APART. BEND AT THE HIPS, KEEP BACK STRAIGHT. LOWER TORSO UNTIL PARALLEL TO FLOOR THEN RETURN TO START. KEEP KNEES SLIGHTLY BENT.

Try this with a weight too

So good
if you sit
alot

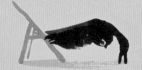

# EXERCISES FOR

# FLEXIBILITY & MOBILITY

Flexibility and mobility exercises help you move better. Keeping your joints healthy and making muscles more stretchy will cut down the risk of injuries and help everyday activities feel easier.

# FORWARD BEND

STAND FACING A CHAIR, FEET
HIP-WIDTH APART. HINGE AT
THE HIPS, PLACE HANDS ON CHAIR
SEAT AND KEEP BACK FLAT.
HOLD, THEN SLOWLY RISE BACK
TO STANDING.

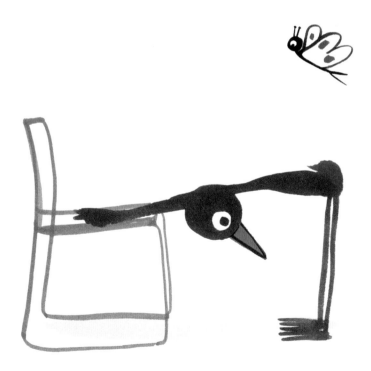

# UPPER-ARM STRETCH

RAISE ONE ARM OVERHEAD,
BEND IT AT THE ELBOW
REACHING DOWN YOUR BACK.
USE OTHER HAND TO GENTLY
PRESS THE ELBOW DOWN.
SWITCH SIDES.

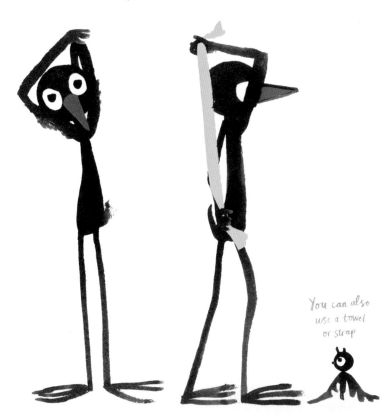

You can also
use a towel
or strap

# SHOULDER STRETCH

BRING RIGHT ARM ACROSS YOUR
UPPER BODY, HOLD IT WITH YOUR
LEFT ARM ABOVE THE ELBOW.
STRETCH AND RELEASE. REPEAT
ON OTHER SIDE.

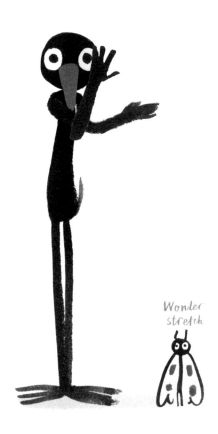

Wonder
stretch

# SEATED TWIST

SIT UPRIGHT ON A CHAIR.
TWIST YOUR TORSO TO THE
LEFT, REST HAND ON THE
CHAIR FOR SUPPORT. HOLD,
THEN RETURN TO CENTRE.
REPEAT ON THE RIGHT.

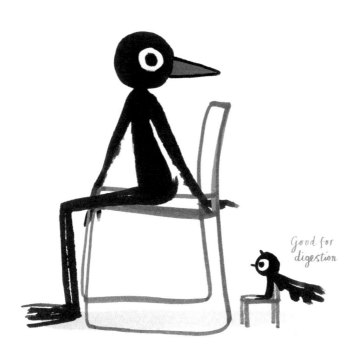

*Good for digestion*

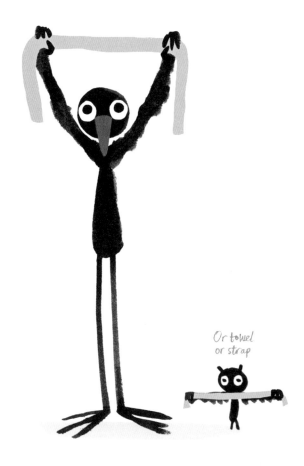

Or towel
or strap

# OVERHEAD ARM STRETCH

HOLD A RESISTANCE BAND IN FRONT OF YOU, WIDER THAN SHOULDERS. LIFT ABOVE HEAD AND WINDMILL BOTH ARMS BEHIND YOU. KEEP ARMS AS STRAIGHT AS POSSIBLE. RETURN TO START AND REPEAT.

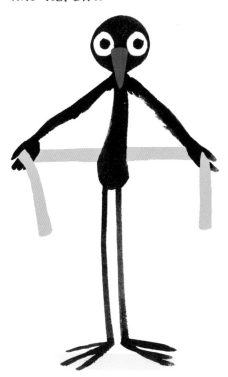

# WARM-UP

Always warm up before exercising to increase the heart rate and blood flow to your muscles. It helps to reduce any stiffness and lowers the risk of injury.

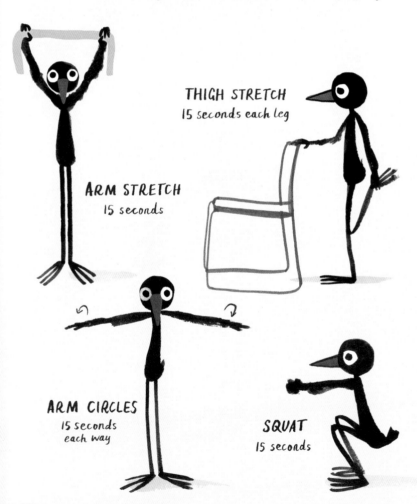

**THIGH STRETCH**
15 seconds each leg

**ARM STRETCH**
15 seconds

**ARM CIRCLES**
15 seconds
each way

**SQUAT**
15 seconds

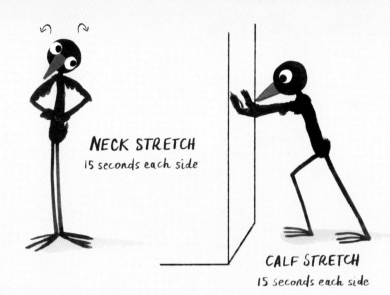

## NECK STRETCH
*15 seconds each side*

## CALF STRETCH
*15 seconds each side*

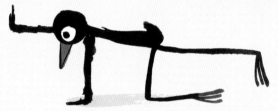

## ARM AND LEG STRETCH
*15 seconds each side*

## PLANK JUMP-IN
*15 seconds*

*I feel warm all over*

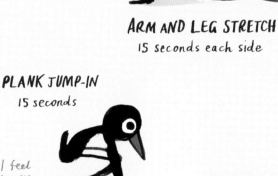

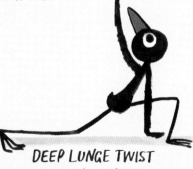

## DEEP LUNGE TWIST
*15 seconds each side*

29

Do you
feel your
heart
pumping?

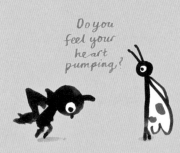

# EXERCISES FOR
# CARDIO

Cardio exercises like running, walking fast and skipping get your heart pumping and the blood flowing. They improve heart and lung function, increasing oxygen supply to your body and muscles.

# STAR JUMPS

START WITH ARMS BY YOUR SIDES, THEN JUMP UP, OPENING ARMS AND LEGS TO MAKE AN 'X' SHAPE. RETURN TO STANDING. REPEAT.

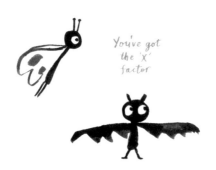

You've got the 'X' factor

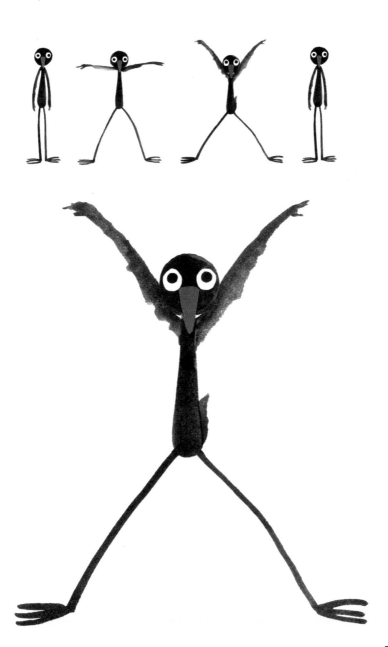

# BURPEES

FROM STANDING, DROP
TO A CROUCH, HANDS TO
FLOOR, JUMP FEET BACK
INTO PLANK, LOWER BODY
TO GROUND, JUMP FEET
TO HANDS, BACK UP TO
STANDING. REPEAT.

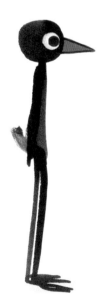
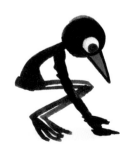
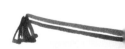

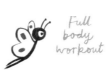

Full
body
workout

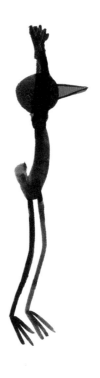

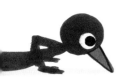

# HIGH KNEES

STAND UPRIGHT, MARCH
ON THE SPOT. LIFT
KNEES AS HIGH AS
POSSIBLE, RAPIDLY
ALTERNATING LEGS.

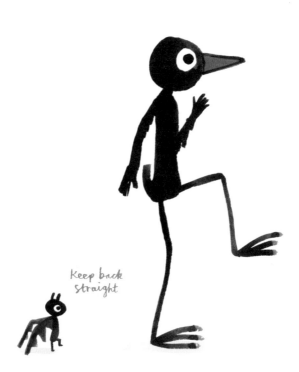

Keep back
straight

# MOUNTAIN CLIMBERS

START IN A PLANK POSITION,
ALTERNATING LEGS, DRAW
ONE KNEE TO YOUR CHEST,
THEN OUT AGAIN. SPEED UP
UNTIL YOU'RE 'RUNNING!'

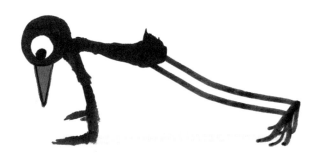

Not for
me

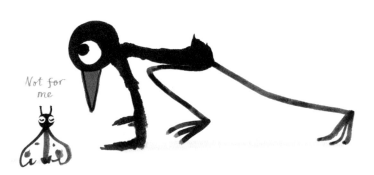

# PLANK JUMP-INS

START IN A PLANK POSITION
AND ENGAGE CORE MUSCLES.
JUMP YOUR FEET TOWARDS
YOUR HANDS THEN BACK
AGAIN, QUICKLY. REPEAT.

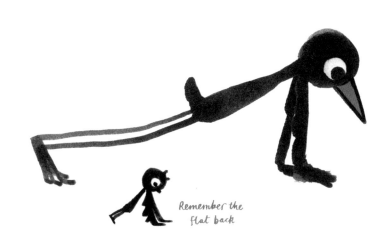

Remember the
flat back

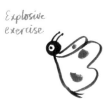

Explosive
exercise

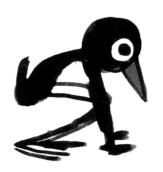

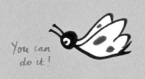

You can
do it!

# EXERCISES FOR

# CORE

Core exercises work the muscles around your tummy, pelvis and back to make your middle section strong. To engage core muscles: breathe out as you pull your naval to spine and draw the internal pelvic muscles upwards at the same time.

# SUPERMAN PRESS

LIE ON YOUR TUMMY AND
ENGAGE CORE MUSCLES.
LIFT ARMS, LEGS AND
CHEST. PULL ELBOWS BACK
AND PRESS SHOULDER
BLADES TOGETHER. EXTEND
ARMS AGAIN AND REPEAT.

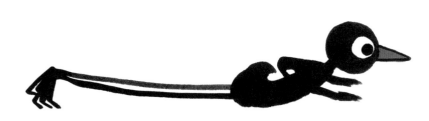

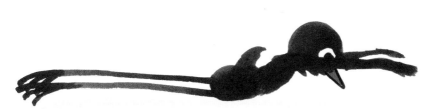

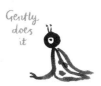

Gently
does
it

# SEATED OBLIQUE TWIST

FROM SITTING, BEND YOUR KNEES AND LEAN BACK TO FORM A 'V' SHAPE. ENGAGE CORE, TWIST RIGHT, RETURN TO CENTRE, THEN TWIST LEFT AND REPEAT.

Raise your feet to make it harder

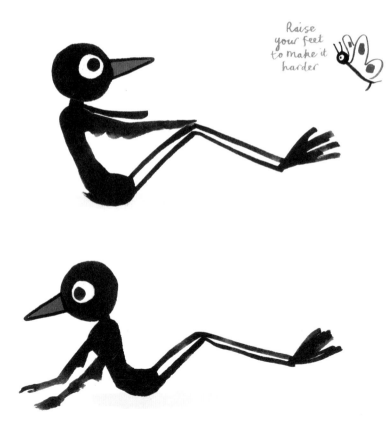

# REVERSE CRUNCH

LIE ON BACK WITH HANDS
BY YOUR SIDE, RAISE LEGS,
PULL KNEES TOWARDS CHEST,
LIFTING HEAD AND HIPS.
LOWER SLOWLY, REPEAT.

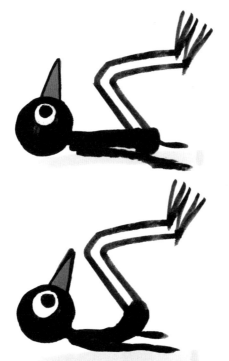

Feel that
in your
tummy

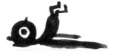

# SIT-UPS

LIE ON YOUR BACK,
KNEES BENT, FEET FLAT
ON FLOOR. ENGAGE CORE
AND RAISE YOUR BODY
TOWARDS THE KNEES
TO SIT UP. LOWER BACK
DOWN AND REPEAT.

Raise your
arms or cross
them over
your chest

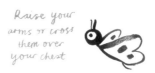

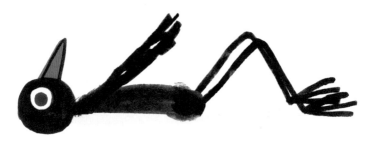

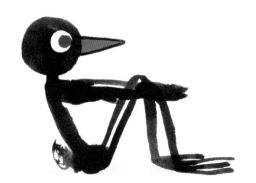

Keep your neck
and shoulders
relaxed

# PLANK

LIE FACE DOWN, PLACE
HANDS UNDER SHOULDERS.
STRAIGHTEN ARMS AND LEGS.
KEEP BODY IN A STRAIGHT
LINE, ENGAGE CORE AND
HOLD POSITION.

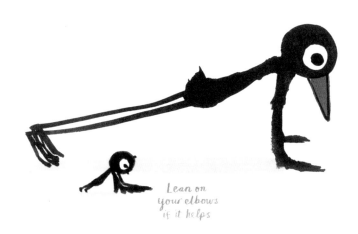

Lean on
your elbows
if it helps

# SIDE PLANK

LIE ON YOUR SIDE, PROP
UP ON ELBOW DIRECTLY
UNDER SHOULDER, STACK
FEET AND HIPS IN A STRAIGHT
LINE FROM HEAD TO FEET.
HOLD, THEN CHANGE SIDES.

If you can
only do one
exercise a day,
the PLANK will
give you the
most benefit

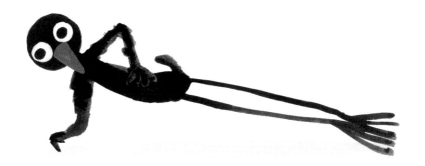

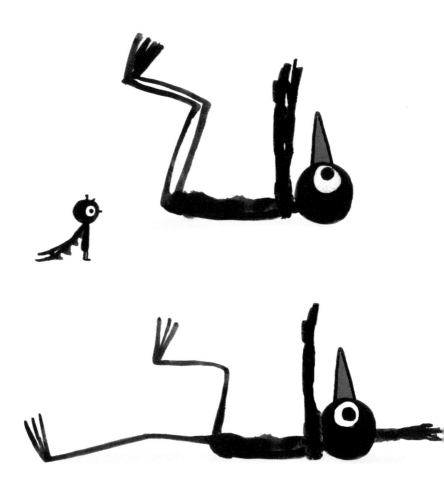

# DEAD BUG

LIE ON YOUR BACK WITH
ARMS AND LEGS UP.
ENGAGE CORE, LOWER
ONE ARM AND THE
OPPOSITE LEG TO FLOOR,
WITH CONTROL. HOVER,
THEN RETURN TO START.
SWITCH SIDES. REPEAT.

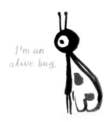

I'm an
alive bug

# BRIDGE POSE

LIE ON BACK WITH FLAT, PARALLEL FEET, HIP-WIDTH APART. KNEES AT RIGHT ANGLE, ARMS BY SIDE, PUSH HIPS UP TO FORM A STRAIGHT LINE FROM SHOULDERS TO KNEES. HOLD, LOWER SLOWLY, REPEAT.

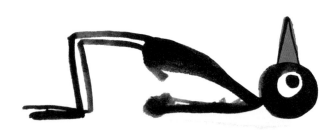

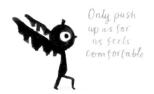

Only push up as far as feels comfortable

# MARCHING BRIDGE

START IN BRIDGE POSE.
LIFT AND LOWER ONE
LEG AT A TIME AS IF
MARCHING. KEEP HIPS
STABLE AND RAISED
THROUGHOUT. REPEAT,
ALTERNATING EACH LEG.

Speed is not
important

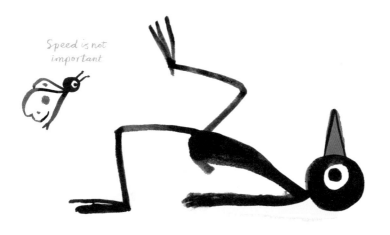

# CARDIO & CORE
# WORKOUT

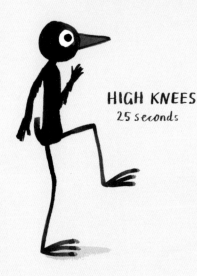

**HIGH KNEES**
*25 seconds*

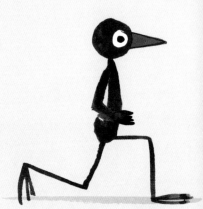

**FORWARD LUNGE**
*25 seconds, alternate legs*

**SIT-UPS**
*25 seconds*

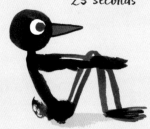

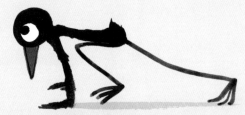

**MOUNTAIN CLIMBER**
*25 seconds, alternate legs*

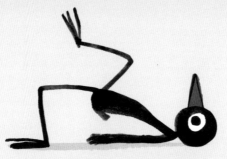

**MARCHING BRIDGE**
25 seconds, alternate legs

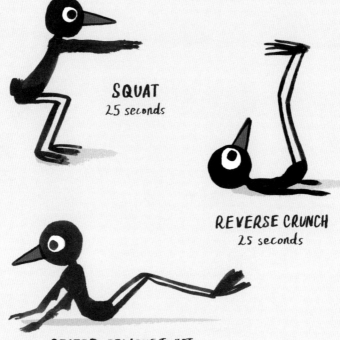

**SQUAT**
25 seconds

**REVERSE CRUNCH**
25 seconds

**SEATED OBLIQUE TWIST**
25 seconds, alternate sides

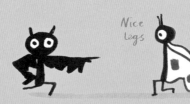

# EXERCISES FOR

# LOWER
## BODY STRENGTH

These exercises strengthen and tone the muscles in the legs and buttocks, improving your balance, stability, coordination and endurance.

# LATERAL LUNGE

STAND WITH FEET PARALLEL
HIP-WIDTH APART. SHIFT
YOUR WEIGHT TO ONE SIDE,
BEND THAT KNEE, KEEPING
OTHER LEG STRAIGHT. PUSH
BACK TO THE START AND
REPEAT ON THE OTHER SIDE.

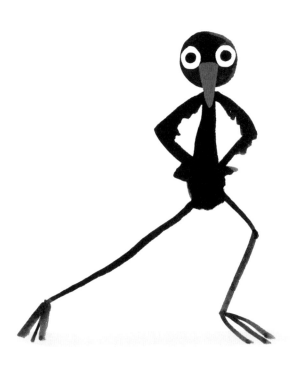

# SIDE LEG RAISE

LIE ON SIDE WITH HIPS AND FEET STACKED. SUPPORT HEAD WITH HAND, ELBOW ON FLOOR. USE OTHER HAND TO PREVENT ROLLING. ENGAGE CORE, LIFT TOP LEG, LOWER SLOWLY. REPEAT WITH OTHER LEG.

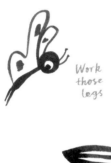

Work those legs

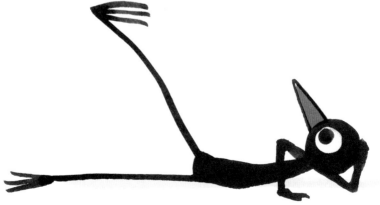

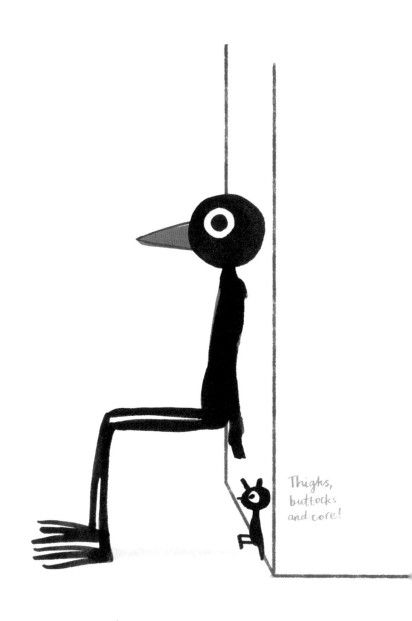

Thighs,
buttocks
and core!

# WALL SIT

LEAN AGAINST A WALL
OR DOOR, SLIDE DOWN
UNTIL YOUR THIGHS ARE
PARALLEL TO THE FLOOR
AND KNEES ARE AT A
RIGHT ANGLE. KEEP BACK
FLAT AND HOLD POSITION.

Makes
my knees
wobble

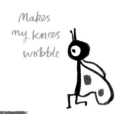

# FIRE HYDRANTS

FROM ALL FOURS, ENGAGE CORE, KEEP BACK FLAT, NECK ALIGNED. WITH ONE KNEE AT A RIGHT ANGLE, MOVE IT OUTWARDS AT 45 DEGREES. LOWER AND REPEAT WITH OTHER LEG.

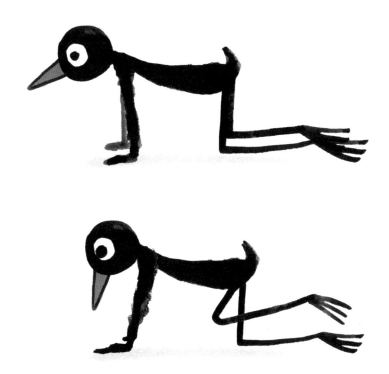

# SQUAT HOLD

LOWER DOWN SLOWLY, HOLD A DEEP SQUAT FOR THREE SECONDS AND PUSH BACK UP FROM YOUR FEET, ENGAGING THE CORE AS YOU RISE TO STANDING.

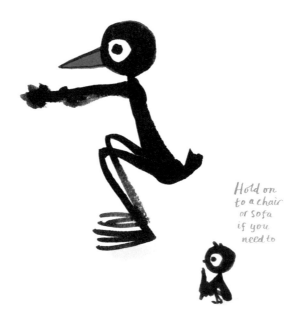

Hold on to a chair or sofa if you need to

# GOBLET SQUAT

STAND WITH FEET HIP-WIDTH APART, HOLD A DUMBBELL CLOSE TO YOUR CHEST, TOP PART IN BOTH HANDS. ELBOWS AT WAIST. ENGAGE CORE, SQUAT. RETURN TO STANDING.

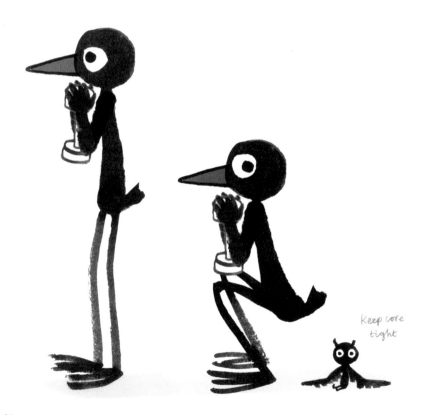

Keep core tight

# CURTSY SQUAT

FROM STANDING, STEP ONE FOOT BACK, HIPS SQUARE, BEND BOTH KNEES TO A RIGHT ANGLE, WEIGHT IN FRONT LEG. HOLD A DUMBBELL IN FRONT OF CHEST. STAND AND SWITCH LEGS.

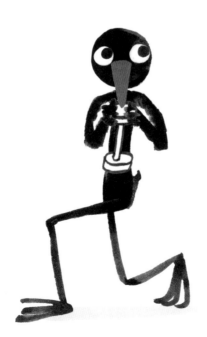

You can do this with or without a weight

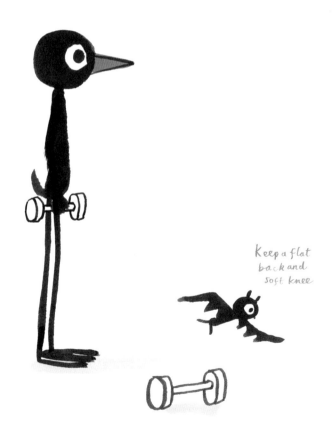

Keep a flat
back and
soft knee

# SINGLE-LEG ROMANIAN DEADLIFT

STAND ON ONE LEG, WITH
(OR WITHOUT) A DUMBBELL
IN OPPOSITE HAND. HINGE AT
THE HIP, EXTEND LEG BEHIND.
LOWER DUMBBELL TOWARDS
GROUND. ENGAGE CORE, STAND
UP. REPEAT ON OTHER SIDE.

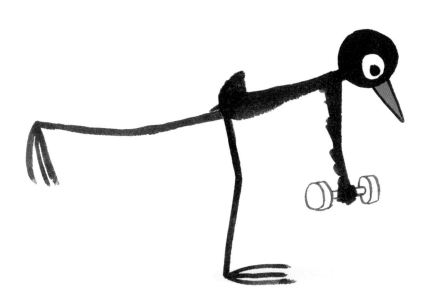

# LOWER-BODY STRENGTH
# WORKOUT

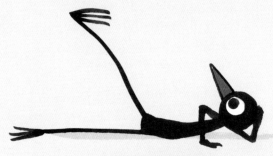

## SINGLE-LEG RAISE
*25 seconds each side*

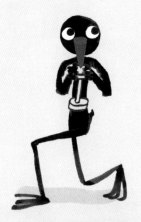

## CURTSY SQUAT
*25 seconds each side*

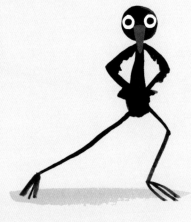

## LATERAL LUNGE
*25 seconds each side*

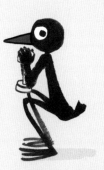

**GOBLET SQUAT**
*25 seconds*

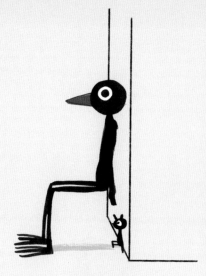

**WALL SIT**
*25 seconds*

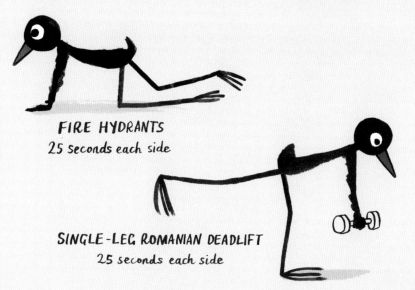

**FIRE HYDRANTS**
*25 seconds each side*

**SINGLE-LEG ROMANIAN DEADLIFT**
*25 seconds each side*

*Up, up
and away*

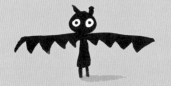

# EXERCISES FOR

# UPPER
# BODY STRENGTH

Working the muscles in the chest,
shoulders and back will improve posture,
enhance upper-body strength and make
it easier to move around in everyday life.

# ARM CIRCLES

STANDING WITH FEET
HIP-WIDTH APART, RAISE
ARMS TO SHOULDER HEIGHT.
ROTATE IN SMALL CIRCLES,
MOVING IN ONE DIRECTION,
THEN THE OTHER.

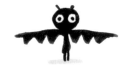

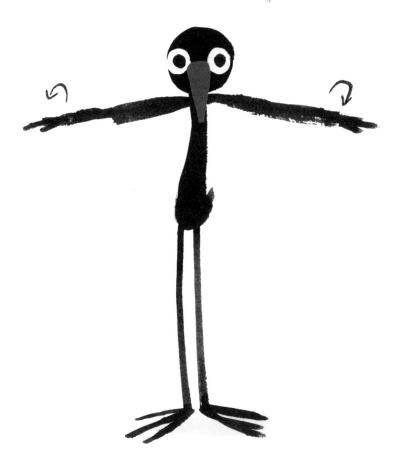

Look straight ahead, feel strong in your core

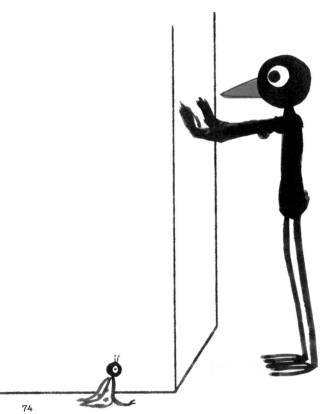

# WALL PUSH-UP

STAND FACING A WALL, PLACE PALMS FLAT ONTO IT, AT WIDTH AND HEIGHT OF SHOULDERS. BEND ELBOWS, LOWER BODY TOWARDS THE WALL. PUSH BACK ON EXHALE. KEEP CORE TIGHT.

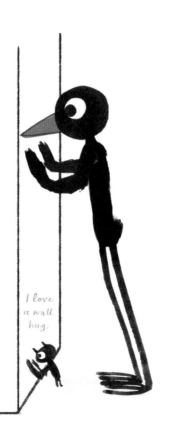

I love a wall hug.

# SHOULDER TAPS

START IN A PLANK POSITION.
RAISE ONE HAND AT A TIME
FROM THE FLOOR TO TAP
THE OPPOSITE SHOULDER.
REPEAT, ALTERNATING HANDS.
AVOID ROCKING AND KEEP
CORE ENGAGED.

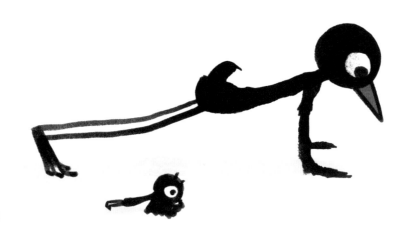

Try it fast
try it slow

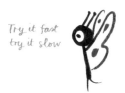

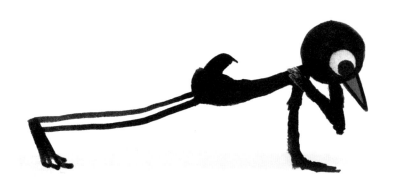

# CHAIR PUSH-UPS

PLACE HANDS ON THE TOP OF A STURDY CHAIR. STEP BOTH FEET BACK, STRAIGHTEN YOUR BODY, SHOULDERS OVER HANDS, LOWER CHEST TOWARDS THE CHAIR. PUSH BACK UP AND REPEAT.

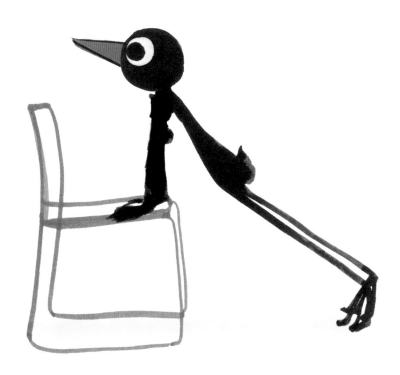

# MINI DIP

SIT ON EDGE OF CHAIR,
LEGS AT A RIGHT ANGLE.
WITH HANDS SUPPORTING
WEIGHT, SLIDE OFF SEAT.
LOWER BODY UNTIL UPPER
ARMS PARALLEL TO FLOOR.
STRAIGHTEN ARMS TO LIFT
BACK UP. REPEAT.

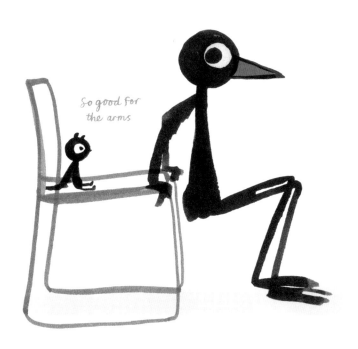

So good for the arms

# UPPER-ARM CURLS

HOLD DUMBBELLS BY YOUR
SIDES, ELBOWS CLOSE. PALMS
FACE BACK. BEND ELBOWS,
CURL WEIGHTS TO SHOULDERS,
LOWER. REPEAT.

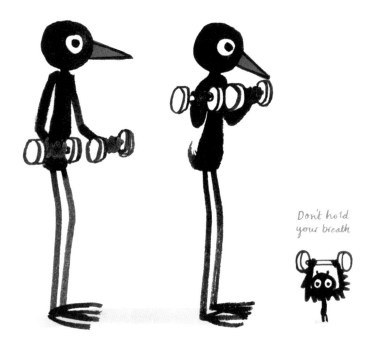

Don't hold
your breath

# ARNOLD PRESS

BEGIN WITH THE UPWARDS
PHASE OF THE UPPER-ARM
CURL. RAISE ARMS OVER
THE HEAD, PALMS FORWARD.
LOWER ARMS AND REPEAT.

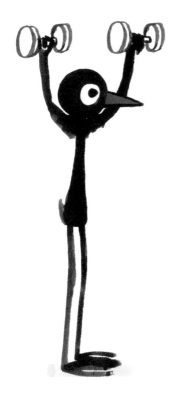

Soft
knees

# UPPER-BODY STRENGTH
# WORKOUT

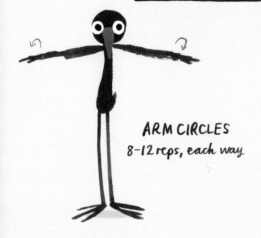

**ARM CIRCLES**
*8-12 reps, each way*

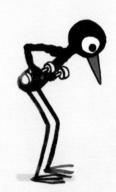

**BENT-OVER ROW**
*8-12 reps*

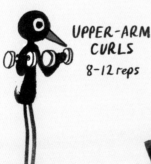

**UPPER-ARM CURLS**
*8-12 reps*

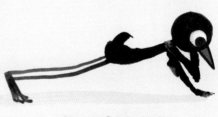

**SHOULDER TAPS**
*8-12 reps*

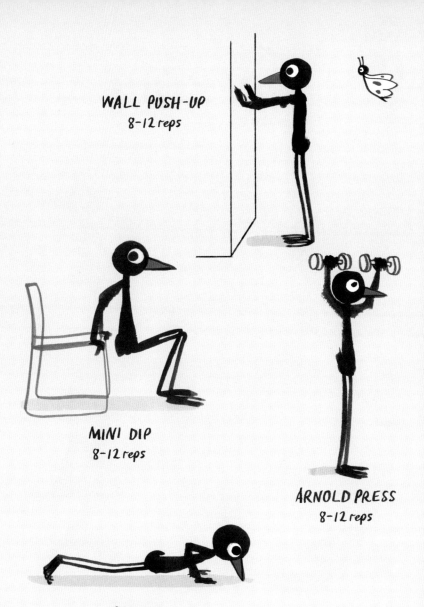

WALL PUSH-UP
8-12 reps

MINI DIP
8-12 reps

ARNOLD PRESS
8-12 reps

PUSH-UP
8-12 reps

83

# 15-MINUTE FULL-BODY
# WORKOUT

Do the whole sequence three times, resting
for one minute between each set.

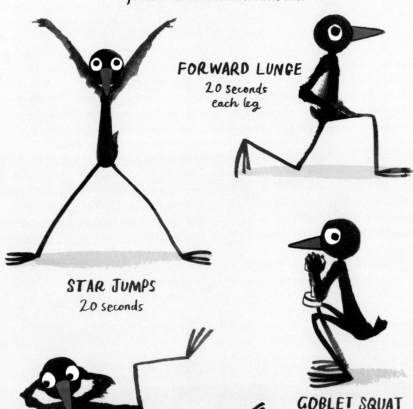

FORWARD LUNGE
20 seconds
each leg

STAR JUMPS
20 seconds

GOBLET SQUAT
20 seconds

BICYCLE CRUNCHES
20 seconds

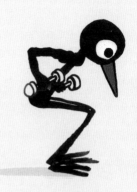

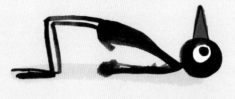

**BRIDGE POSE**
8–12 reps

**BENT-OVER ROW**
8–12 reps

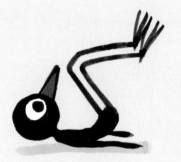

**REVERSE CRUNCH**
20 seconds

**SHOULDER TAPS**
8–12 reps

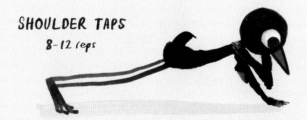

# COOL-DOWN

Cooling down after a workout is great for getting your heart rate back to normal, speeding up recovery, easing muscle soreness and cutting down on injuries. It also makes you more flexible.

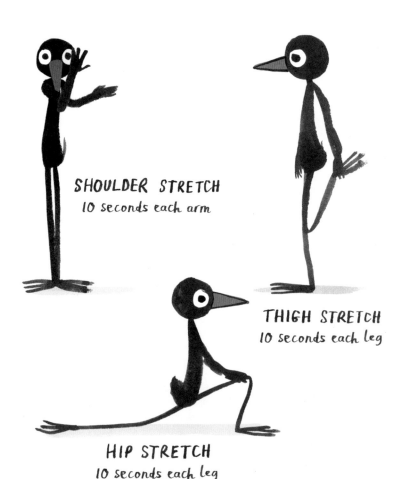

**SHOULDER STRETCH**
10 seconds each arm

**THIGH STRETCH**
10 seconds each leg

**HIP STRETCH**
10 seconds each leg

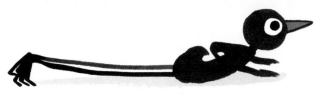

**BACK EXTENSION**
10 seconds

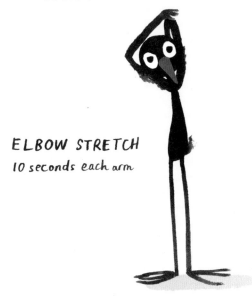

**ELBOW STRETCH**
10 seconds each arm

*I do like
a good
cool down*

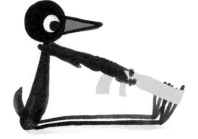

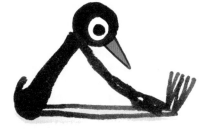

**SEATED FORWARD BEND**
10 seconds

THANK YOU TO ZARA LARCOMBE, ROLY ALLEN,
VIRGINIA BREHAUT, ALISON GUILE, ANGUS HYLAND,
VANESSA GREEN AT THE URBAN ANT, FELICITY AWDRY,
NATALIA PRICE-CABRERA AND ELIZABETH SHEINKMAN PFD.

**Skittledog**

FIRST PUBLISHED IN THE UNITED KINGDOM IN 2025 BY SKITTLEDOG,
AN IMPRINT OF THAMES & HUDSON LTD, 181A HIGH HOLBORN,
LONDON WC1V 7QX

HOW TO BE A FIT BIRD © 2025 THAMES & HUDSON LTD, LONDON

TEXT AND ILLUSTRATIONS © M. DEUCHARS LTD 2025

BRITISH LIBRARY CATALOGUING-IN-PUBLICATION DATA
A CATALOGUE RECORD FOR THIS BOOK IS AVAILABLE FROM
THE BRITISH LIBRARY

ISBN 978-1-837-76050-3

PRINTED AND BOUND IN CHINA BY C&C OFFSET PRINTING CO., LTD

MIX
Paper | Supporting
responsible forestry
FSC® C008047
FSC
www.fsc.org

BE THE FIRST TO KNOW ABOUT OUR NEW RELEASES,
EXCLUSIVE CONTENT AND AUTHOR EVENTS BY VISITING
SKITTLEDOG.COM
THAMESANDHUDSON.COM
THAMESANDHUDSONUSA.COM
THAMESANDHUDSON.COM.AU